DEFEATING DRUGS AND DEATH

HOW TO STOP DRUG ADDICTION

ANTHONY EKANEM

ISBN 978-1-63997-709-3

Contents

Preface

Drugs are chemicals that can change the way the human body works. If you have ever been sick and had to take medication, you already have an idea about drugs. Medicines are drugs doctors prescribe to patients. But do you know that even medicines prescribed by doctors can be dangerous if they are not taken as prescribed?

Some drugs are dangerous to human health all the time. Doctors do not prescribe or give these drugs to their patients. Alcohol and cigarettes are included in this class of drugs. Even if people can buy them legally at pharmacy stores, they can be dangerous to health. Illegal drugs are very harmful, and they include cocaine, marijuana, heroin and ecstasy.

DIFFERENT KINDS OF DRUGS

You have read that drugs can be harmful to you. But why are they bad? And what does that mean? Listed below are the various types of drugs you should be aware of and how they affect an individual's life:

MEDICINES – THE LEGAL DRUGS

If you had been sick and you took medication to get better, you already know this kind of drugs. Medicines are legal drugs and doctors give them to patients. A pharmacy store may also sell them, and individuals can buy them across the counter. However, it is not safe for you to take medicines without a doctor's prescription or buy them from people who sell them illegally.

ALCOHOL AND CIGARETTES

Cigarettes and alcohol are other types of legal drugs. In many countries of the world, people who are 18 years and above can buy them. Note, however, that excessive drinking and smoking are very dangerous to health.

ILLEGAL DRUGS

When people talk about drugs problems, they mean abusing legal or illegal drugs. Generally, cannabis is an illegal drug. However, due to some health benefits that it can bring, some countries permit doctors to prescribe it to adults for certain ailments.

Drugs do not solve problems. Using drugs could cause other issues aside from the problems you had already. Somebody who is using these could become addicted. This just means that the body of the person may become so accustomed to having this drug that he or she cannot do without it.

Once you are addicted to these drugs, it can be very difficult to stop taking them. Discontinuing the use of the drugs can cause withdrawal symptoms, which may include sweating, tremors and vomiting. These feelings can continue until the body can adjust to being free from drugs again.

HOW TO KNOW SOMEONE WHO USES DRUGS

If an individual is using illegal drugs, you may notice changes in the person's actions or looks. Below are some of the signs of someone who uses or abuses drugs. It is important to know that depression or other issues could also cause such changes in an individual.

Someone who uses drugs:

- Will hang out with other drugs users
- Would be negative, worried, or moody most of the time
- Wants to be alone most of the time
- Cannot concentrate
- Sleeps every time
- Gains or loses weight

- Have runny nose all the time
- Coughs a lot
- Have puffy or red eyes

TERMS RELATING TO DRUGS

- **Addiction.** Someone is experiencing addiction if they are always dependent on drugs.

- **Depressant.**Depressants are drugs that slow a person down. Doctors prescribe depressants to help people to be less anxious, angry or tense. Depressants can also relax the muscles and make someone feel less stressed or sleepy. Several individuals can also illegally use such drugs to slow themselves down as well as help them to sleep, particularly after using different types of stimulants.

- **Stimulant.**Stimulants speed up the brain and body. Some of these are cocaine and methamphetamines. These are opposite of depressants. Naturally, stimulants can energise people and make them feel high. When the effects of stimulants wear off, a person will feel sick or tired.

- **Narcotic.**Narcotic drugs dull the human senses and relieve pains. They can cause an individual to get into the stupor, sleep, coma, or convulsions. Narcotics like codeine can be legal if prescribed by doctors in treating pains. Heroin is another illegal narcotic drug with side effects, and it can be very addictive.

- **Hallucinogen.**Hallucinogen is a drug like LSD, which

changes the mood of the person and makes him or her hear or see things that are not there or think of some strange things.

- **High.** This is the feeling that drug users like to experience when taking hard drugs. There are many kinds of highs, including a spacey feeling.

- **Inhalant.**Like gasoline or glue, once sniffed could provide users with an immediate rush. Inhalants produce a feeling of drunkenness, which can cause the individual to stagger, get confused, and some feelings of sleepiness and dizziness.

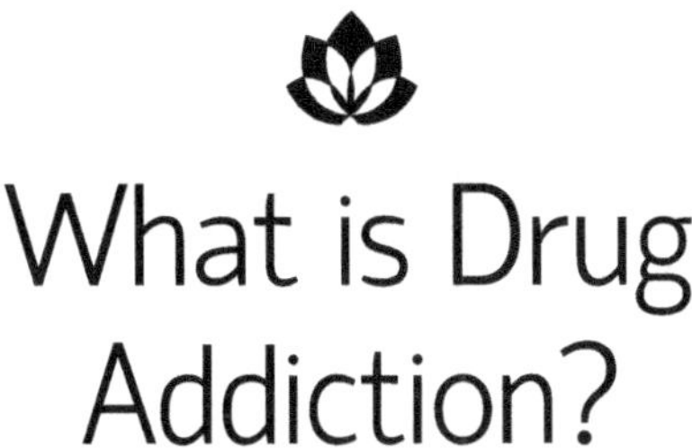

CHAPTER ONE

What is Drug Addiction?

Drug addiction is a severe problem, and it is not only found in certain areas or with certain types of people. Addiction is found everywhere and with all kinds of people. It does not matter if an individual is rich or poor, male or female, strong or weak or what part of the world they live in, addiction is real. That is why it is so important that you are well informed about addiction. This is because no matter who you are or where you live, if you make poor decisions involving drugs, addiction is waiting just around the corner.

People can be misled about drug use and addiction, either because they have spoken to the wrong people or because they have not talked to anyone at all about it. This is quite understandable. It can be difficult to talk to people about drug abuse and addiction, particularly when the person affected is already going down the slippery slope of drug abuse and addiction.

Being ensnared in drug addiction or knowing someone with an addiction problem can feel as if you are sucked into a deep hole with no hope of coming out, and death waiting just at the other end of the tunnel. Those who are currently experiencing addiction or are now in recovery know how true that statement is. The worst part of drug addiction is that once it has become full-blown, it makes people delusional about how bad their problem is.

Convincing somebody about how much they have damaged their body can be likened to trying to reason with a rock: they don't just listen. In many cases, it is not until the addict reaches their lowest point in life, that they begin to see what their life has become. Sadly, this point is often sooner followed by death.

Drug addiction comes in different forms. There are mental and physical drug addictions. Mental addictions are severe, but it can be easier to deal with than physical addictions. This is because physical addiction stems from a lack of chemicals produced in the brain because of drug abuse.

Chemicals that are naturally produced by the body to regulate the mood and energy levels are produced at a slower rate when drugs are taken regularly. This is to compensate for the dopamine and serotonin that the brain receptors are trying to take in. At first, these chemicals in the brain will cause ecstatic feelings, but as time passes, the brain starts to produce less of the chemicals. This brings about more drug use and subsequent addiction.

The use of more drugs to reach the same level of euphoria is known as "chasing the high". Ultimately, this makes it difficult for the brain to produce relevant chemicals, and the person becomes depressed without the drug. The affected individual could have difficulty functioning without using the drug and can become bodily ill as a result. Good examples of physically addictive drugs include heroin and alcohol. Both drugs can make the user feel sick, and that is why most users of heroin and alcohol must go through a detox process before going for rehabilitation.

If you are a parent and you are trying to prevent your child or loved ones from using illegal drugs, the following are some tips that can help you in your effort.

KNOW THEIR FRIENDS

You must know all their friends. You need to sit down and talk with their friends to know the type of personS they are. A lot of parents know the names of their children's friends but do not know anything about them. This can create a very risky situation as most children start using drugs following the influence of their social and peer groups. This is especially true around the junior high to the high school phases of the child's life.

BE INVOLVED IN THEIR LIFE

Everyone wants to feel loved, so it is imperative to get involved in your child's daily life. Do all you can to show them that you care about them. It may be difficult at times to make time for this, but it is crucial and should be thought of as your top priority.

BE HONEST AND HAVE DISCUSSIONS

This is probably the most critical step you need to take to prevent or treat addiction. If your loved ones cannot confide in you, they will most likely stray off in different directions. You can avoid this by being open with your loved ones and letting know they can confide in you.

CHAPTER TWO

Accept That You Need Help

Accepting the fact that you need help when fighting an addiction can be very challenging. This process is often made difficult as a result of the irrational state of mind of drug addicts who no longer see reality for what it is. Instead of seeing the damage that they cause to themselves, they would only see the "positives" that they think the drug is giving them.

If you are eager to get rid of your addiction, the first and possibly the most important step is to admit the fact that you have a problem and you need help. Being honest with yourself will help make your situation better.

It is understandable why some people find it difficult to come to terms with how their addiction has become out-of-control. It is mentally hard to accept that fact, and that can cause an individual to feel depressed or feel like a failure when they see how bad things have become.

Even though it can be difficult, and sometimes painful, this step is necessary if you want to overcome your addiction. This is the very first step in almost all addiction recovery programmes. In looking at the steps, you will discover that step one is to admit that you are helpless as regards your addiction. This does not mean that you can do nothing to stop your addiction. It means that you do not control your addiction; your addiction controls you, and you will need help in the process of recovery.

This process can be carried out with a drug therapist or sponsor. Some people may accept this reality clandestinely because the truth might be difficult to accept, and they don't want to burst around other people emotionally. No matter how you choose to do this, it must get done. You will not be able to overcome your drug addiction if you don't admit that you have a problem.

Some people may continually refuse to accept the truth. These individuals who don't leave the denial stage will likely not recover from their addiction and may die from their illegal drug use. Stop your drug addiction and accept the fact that you have a problem and you need help before it is too late.

CHAPTER THREE

Drug Detox Basics

As mentioned before, some addictions will require the addict to go to a detox clinic before starting a rehabilitation programme. This is because withdrawal from some types of hard drugs can make them ill or even kill them.

A common type of addiction that can result in this is alcoholism. It is important to know the facts about detoxification and what an individual may experience while going through a detox programme. It is advisable that, if available in your area, you go to a detoxification clinic and don't do a detox by yourself. It is good to be supervised by trained professionals to forestall any medical problems.

KNOW WHAT TO EXPECT

To be honest with you, detoxification will not be an easy process. You will likely experience different side effects of your drug use. The side effects could be emotional, mental or physical. You may experience various uncomfortable feelings. In other words, you may not feel great about life during the detox process, but it is crucial for recovery.

The following are examples of what you may go through during a detox process:

SWEATS, CHILLS, VOMITING:

You may experience these side effects while detoxifying, depending on the drugs you were addicted to. As stated before, heroin and alcohol addiction normally have these types of side effects when detoxifying.

If you are going through this process at home instead of a clinic, which is not advisable, you need to make sure that you hydrate yourself. Even though you know that you cannot keep liquids down, you must keep drinking water. This is because you need to replace all the fluid you lose from sweating. Another reason you should do your detoxification in a clinic is that they can give you medications to make you feel good. A drug commonly prescribed for heroin abusers is methadone. You must be careful with this drug because it can also be addictive.

MOOD CHANGES

Detoxifying from a drug can have significant impacts on someone's mood. A person who is always happy, or appears to be happy because they are *high*, can turn to be in a different mood. They could become cantankerous and snap at people for no clear reason, or they can feel depressed and reason that life is no longer worth living.

It is imperative to show sympathy and compassion to someone who is going through this type of painful experience. Although it may be difficult to deal with their attitude, you can take comfort in knowing that you are helping them to overcome their problem. If you are the one going through the detoxification process, try not to take it out on people as mood changes are common.

CRAVING

Craving is another side effect of drug addiction. When someone is in the process of detoxifying, they may have some strong cravings. Some drugs produce stronger cravings than others. So, depending on the addiction an individual is suffering, it could be a moderate craving or one that controls their thoughts.

The way to get over this is to distract yourself when you feel a craving. You can call a friend and have a chat with them or do some other things that can take your attention away from drug use. Although cravings can feel as if they will not go away, they will, and they get less often over time.

There are positive outcomes from detoxifying, and the following are a few examples:

BETTER HEALTH

Although you might feel terrible in the early stages of detoxification, your overall health will be improving. You will notice your natural complexion coming back while the dark circles will be leaving your eyes. You will feel better and more energetic than before.

MENTAL AND EMOTIONAL STATE

You will notice that you begin thinking clearer and that things begin to make more sense. This is because your mind is no longer being filled with the cloud of fog that addiction was causing. Also, your emotional state will improve, and you will be better able to handle situations in life reasonably.

LESS STRESS FOR LOVED ONES

Your loved ones will appreciate the fact that you have decided to get help, beginning with detoxifying. This will put their minds at rest as they will no longer live in fear of losing you. You can imagine how it would feel to have this concern for your child and other people you care about. It would be frightening.

BETTER SELF-ESTEEM

Detoxification will boost your self-esteem. You will feel as if you can walk tall and hold your head high once a substance is no longer ruling you. Not only will you be proud of yourself, but those who are close to you will be proud of you too. It will feel better when the people who know you see that you are recovering and are no longer taking drugs. They will be filled with joy and pride as opposed to fear, concern, and disapproval.

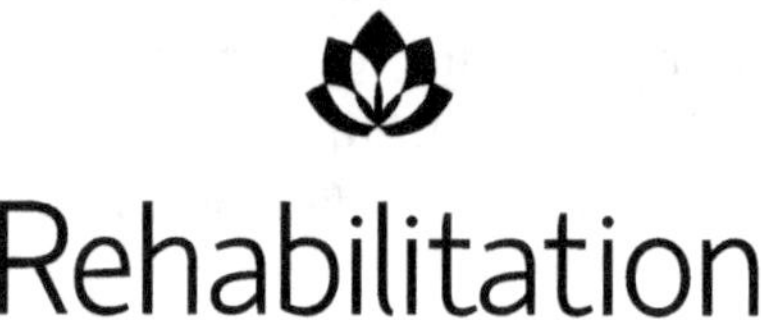

CHAPTER FOUR

Rehabilitation

Even though the thought of going to rehabilitation could be frightening, it is necessary for recovery. In many cases, drug addicts may not overcome all the difficulties associated with their addiction. They must turn to professional help in a rehabilitation facility. There are different types of rehabilitation with varying levels of treatment.

Most rehabilitation centres have an unlocked room door policy but lock the doors that enter and exit the facility. There is a possibility that you may need to share a room with other patients while in specific rehabilitation centres. If this is the case with you, make sure to check their policy on it first. There are also rehabilitation centres with lock-down facilities. These are equivalent to prisons, and most people in such facilities were ordered by the courts to be there.

Once you enter a rehabilitation centre, you will meet with a drug counsellor. They will figure out your specific addiction issues and come up with a treatment plan. They will take your medical history and do a check-up on you. During your stay at the facility, your medication will be kept with the nurse who will also dispense them to you as the needs arise. This is done to forestall any attempt on your part to abuse your medication.

You will have counselling and group therapy sessions that you will be required to attend regularly. There could also be sporting events or outings that you may be expected to attend. All this is intended to provide you with the best treatment and help possible.

You must be honest with your counsellors at the rehabilitation centre. Do not be in a hurry to go back home. Being dishonest with your counsellors to return home quicker could lead to failure in your battle with addiction. Although it is not easy to be away from home for an extended period, it is in your best interest to remain in rehabilitation until your counsellors deem it fit to let you go. This is the only way you can be sure of a better future, a healthy life, and good relationships.

If in-patient rehabilitation is not an option for you, there are rehabilitation centres that offer out-patient treatments. You must be careful if you decide to go for this option because it does not prevent you from obtaining drugs that can still put you at risk. Many rehabilitation centres have follow-up programmes for addicts that have been discharged.

CHAPTER FIVE

Nutrition for Recovering Addicts

A large part of winning in your battle with addiction is to have a proper diet. You may find it difficult to believe this, but it is true. While you are trying to gain control of your addiction, you must have a balanced diet and avoid too much sugar and caffeine. It is advisable to look up the food pyramid as you prepare your meals.

PREPARE A PROPER DIET

It is important that while in recovery you eat a proper dict. This will make you feel good and healthy. When you feel very good, you will have less craving to use drugs to "feel good". Drug addiction takes a severe toll on human health. Therefore, you must eat well to regain your strength and good health.

Studies have shown that specific diets can help an addict with their recovery. These studies state that the daily diet of a recovering addict should include:

- **30% Fat**
- **25% Protein**
- **45% Carbohydrates**

It is important to remember that like anything else, these foods are good in moderation. For instance, fruits are very healthy, but too much fruit can be bad. Also, just because chicken is healthy does not mean you should have a plateful of chicken for dinner. Eat everything in moderation.

You must avoid excessive sugar and caffeine. They are stimulants. They can mimic the effect of some drugs which can cause triggers in some individuals.

If you smoke, another part of your recovery diet is to quit smoking. A lot of people do not know that nicotine is a stimulant. Just like caffeine, nicotine can cause triggers. The smoke can remind you of using a drug and make you have a craving.

CHAPTER SIX

Effects of Drug Addiction

If you are the one struggling with drug addiction, or know a friend or loved one who is, then you must be aware that it slowly deteriorates everything in the life of the addict. It begins with smaller unnoticeable things, and before long, your entire world is turned upside down. If you are curious about what drug addiction can ultimately lead to, this chapter has the answers you may be looking for.

WHAT WILL HAPPEN

Numerous things can happen from drug addiction, and none of them is positive. The adverse consequences of drug addiction are numerous. Listed below are examples of what may happen to you if you are a drug addict.

1. **Loss of Relationships**

Everyone has a breaking point. This means that no matter how someone may love you, there get to a point where they can no longer take the stress and they are forced to part ways. This may likely fuel addiction more and make things even worse. Sometimes it ends in suicide or other terrible consequences.

2. Going to Jail

As a drug addict, it may not be very long before you are arrested by law enforcement agencies who are already tired of hard and illegal drugs issues. They are meting out stiffer penalties, even to first-time offenders to serve as a deterrent. Having drug charges on your record will add complications to your financial situation since getting a good job would be very difficult.

3. Sexually Transmitted Diseases

Some drug use may lead to the contraction of STDs, especially drugs that are injected. The rate of people with sexually transmitted diseases and Hepatitis C is very high. Many drug addicts do not care about their hygiene and safety. They share needles and other sharp objects in addition to having unprotected sex with people they should not.

4. Death

An addiction can eventually lead to death. It does not matter how much a person thinks they are in control; they are delusional! Abusing drugs slowly kills addicts and damages the health of those who care for them due to the high stress of the situation. You must begin recovery!

CHAPTER SEVEN

The Gains of Being Drug-Free

For a lot of people, stopping the use of illegal and hard drugs is not the most difficult aspect of getting rid of addiction. Living drug-free or alcohol-free is the most challenging aspect. There are many reasons for this, one of which is that some people feel pains when withdrawing from the drugs. Such pains can be the cause of abandonment, child abuse and abnormal sexual relations, or the loss of a loved one. There are not easy problems, but this can be harder if combined with the issue of recovering from drugs and alcohol.

No matter your reasons for using drugs or alcohol, try to be alcohol and drug-free. Once you can stop using drugs or alcohol, you will experience many benefits which you have not thought of.

Living a drug-free life can provide more freedom compared to the artificial feeling of freedom you can get from being high. Drug users may try escaping through addiction. They may be stressed after work and then use drugs to relax. Addiction does not provide a solution or healing. It cannot also give the benefits of living a drug-free life, which may include the following:

THE FAMILY

One of the essential aspects of living a drug-free life is the family aspect. Drug addiction or abuse could tear families apart. Drug use can cause mood swings, violence, cheating and financial difficulties. There are not many families that may remain strong during drug addiction while a drug-free life can heal a family.

STRESS MANAGEMENT

Even though a lot of people feel that drug use takes away stress, addiction and abuse have the opposite effect. Once you become dependent on drugs, the mere thought of not being able to take another one can be stressful. Trying to take more drugs or hiding drug use from your loved ones, coupled with financial stress, can be overbearing. No matter where you live in the world, being drug-free is the best life to live.

YOUR CAREER

Living a drug-free life will let you excel and keep your job. Some drug users find it difficult to focus or care about their job. In addition to that, addiction could also get you fired. You are not only harming yourself, but also other people around you.

MENTAL STABILITY

Several drugs can cause mental health problems, and these may lead to addiction. Once this starts, it will require expert help and hard work to stop. Living a drug-free life will provide you with much-needed mental health and stability.

YOUR WELLBEING

Your general wellbeing will be affected once you abuse any drug. This includes your relationships, values, priorities and physical health. Living a drug-free life will benefit you in every aspect of your life.

There are countless other benefits you will enjoy from being drug-free. If you do not want to ruin your life and your relationship, then do not hesitate to get rid of illegal drugs. There are better things you could do with your life. You don't need to take hard drugs to get rid of any issues or problems. Drugs are not solutions to any problem. They can only give you momentary false relief after which they will ruin your life in the long run.

LIFE WITHOUT ALCOHOL

For some people, not drinking alcohol could be a difficult task. Though alcohol is not prohibited for people who are 18 years and above in most countries of the world, it is always wise to drink moderately. Addiction to alcohol is dangerous and can destroy everything you have already accomplished.

Abstinence from alcohol can give you a healthy body and a cheerful mind. You will not have to deal with hangovers. Getting off any bad habit will assist you in sustaining a positive outlook, useful decisions, and a better life. Your work will improve. Your relationships will improve, so also is your mindset. Overall, abstinence from alcohol will benefit you in many ways. Below are a few of them:

HEALTHY LIVER

One of the numerous functions of the liver is alcohol's assimilation. The majority of alcoholic drinks that you consume is absorbed and metabolized into the body through the liver. This organ of the body can only process a half-ounce of alcohol each hour. If you have consumed more, the liver will not be able to handle it, and complications can arise. Moreover, if this goes unchecked for some time, your liver can be damaged permanently. You may also suffer from other liver disorders.

SHARPER BRAIN

Because of alcohol, brain cells can be affected. Using too much alcohol could result in lesions on one's brain. This can also damage the reasoning functions and memory. Those who are addicted to alcohol can sometimes lose their ability to maintain long-term memory. Because of the alcohol inhibition effect, this has been linked with increased domestic violence, child abuse, and adolescent pregnancies. On the other hand, teetotalers always maintain a grasp of themselves and are responsible for their actions.

SOUND HEART

Even if moderate wine consumption is renowned for reducing the risks of various heart ailments, most alcoholic beverages have higher contents of alcohol compared to wine. That is why you should live an alcohol-free life.

IMPROVED SEX LIFE

Prolonged alcohol abuse and addiction may cause hormonal imbalance. This can result in estrogen hypersecretion which can lead to impotence or erectile dysfunction in men. Abstinence from alcohol can stabilise hormone levels.

REDUCED RISK OF CANCER

The hormonal imbalance that causeS impotence in men may lead to breast cancer in women. Alcohol has also been linked with different ailments of the pancreas like pancreatic cancer.

SAFER PREGNANCIES FOR WOMEN

The placental barrier between the mother and her baby is permeable to the alcohol. If the pregnant woman consumes the drink, the fetus can be invariably affected. This can lead to miscarriages, congenital disorders or stillbirth. Even though you are not a teetotaler, alcohol must not be taken when you are pregnant. Not drinking alcohol can put a woman at lesser risk when they are pregnant so they can avoid medical complications.

AVOID OBESITY

Alcohol contains more sugar compared to fruits. This can lead to unhealthy weight gain. Obesity increases the chances of having severe health problems, such as diabetes, depression, and heart problems. It is very difficult to reduce the weight gained through alcohol use.

BETTER SLEEP

Alcohol is a depressant and can cause drowsiness. It disturbs sleep patterns, particularly in your sleep's second half. Having a good night's sleep can make you very productive. And this can be useful in your career, especially if you have busy schedules.

IMPROVED SOCIAL LIFE

Alcohol addiction can also lead to social and psychological problems. As mentioned earlier, excessive alcohol intake can cause hormonal imbalance which can cause insomnia, depression, dementia, and so on. If you stop taking too much alcohol, you can get rid of mental or psychological issues. And that can make you live a better social life. If you find it difficult to live a drug and alcohol-free life on your own, there is nothing to worry about. You can always rely on professionals to provide you with services that can make your life better. Once you have successfully gotten rid of drug and alcohol addiction, you will be able to enjoy all the benefits mentioned above, and so much more.